The Role of Pastoral Caregivers to the Terminally Ill Patients

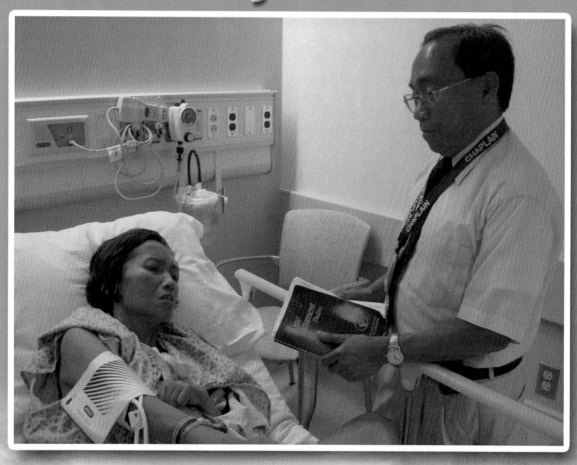

A RESOURCE MANUAL

Jim E. Garcines

Print information available on the last page

Rev. Date: 02/15/2016

To order additional copies of this book, contact:
Xlibris
1-888-795-4274
www.Xlibris.com
Orders@Xlibris.com

Jim E. Garcines provides a brief overview of a pastor's duties in ministering to the terminally ill in this slim and insightful manual.

Originally from Cagayan de Oro City in the Philippines, Garcines moved to California in 1983 and began a church in San Jose two years later. This resource manual is the culmination of Garcines' chaplaincy work, where he was "the first one absorbing all the agonies, regrets, failures, misery, anger and hurts" of dying patients. He brings his experiences and expertise together in this short offering.

Garcines examines the stages and responses that are most commonly seen in dying patients and their family members. He encourages pastors to be "positive without expecting that you are going to cheer them up. Be prepared for their feeling of depression…your job is to be a manifestation of God's love for and presence to them." Garcines shows that ministering to the terminally ill must be handled with delicate care, as circumstances vary greatly from patient to patient.

A portion of the manual is dedicated to the experiences and perspectives of medical professionals at UC Davis Medical Center in Sacramento, CA. He includes their comments and answers to questions regarding patients' reactions to the news that they are dying, how these professionals cope with the stress of caring for the terminally ill, tips for handling hostility from family members, and more.

This manual will be eye opening for anyone who has never worked in this field or has had yet to confront the realities of death. While the information could certainly be expanded and each subject explored further and more deeply, Garcines' humble nature and sincere concern for dying patients is clearly evident. His heartfelt and sober book can serve as a useful initiation for those new to the care of the terminally ill.

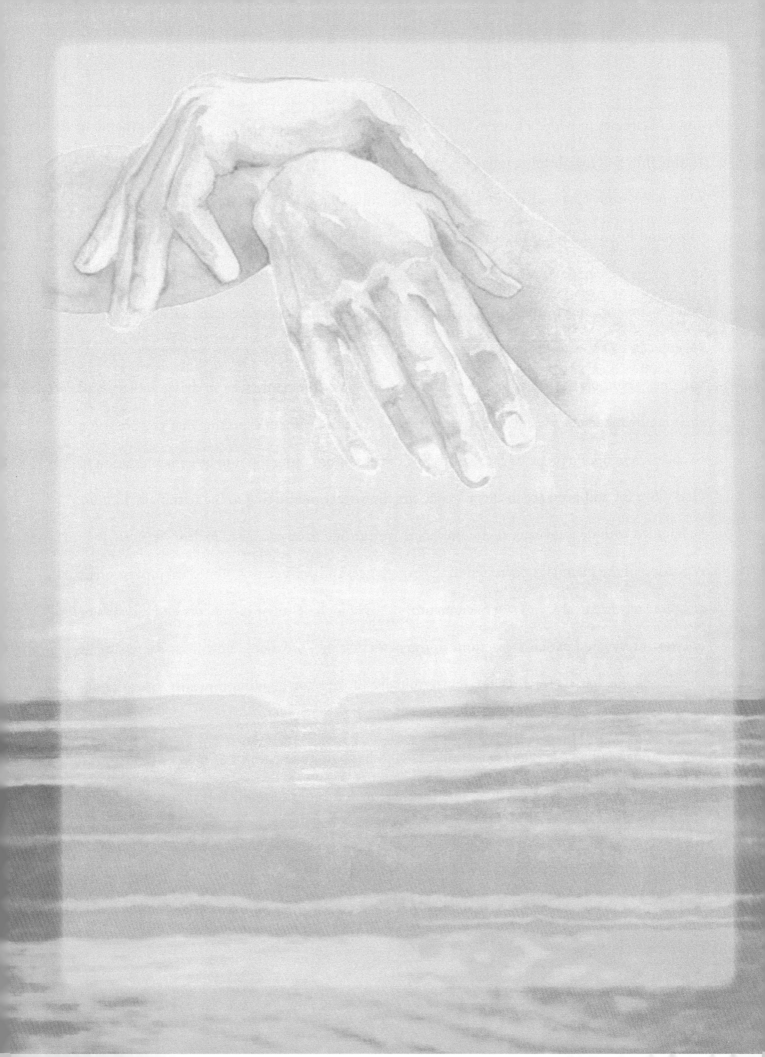

To my dearest wife, Carol, who taught, encouraged and inspired my tough journey with God. She was a great help as I write this manual . She is a godly woman, a mentor whose life immensely touch's lives as she teaches children, parents and women in our church. But above all she raised our two children in the path of God.

- Jim

I. Introduction

I am privileged to have great opportunity to work in the hospital where I had been exposed to and experienced several needs in pastoral care. I had visited countless patients each day as I do my rounds to various departments in varied situations and conditions as well as responding to Code Blue. My daily experiences had taught me a lot on how to effectively minister to patients who are terminally ill and dying. Several times, I feel hurt and sympathetic together with the family of patients. I am the first one absorbing all the agonies, regrets, failures, misery, anger, and hurts of the patients as they share what they are going through in their conditions, which taught me to be a more humble, compassionate, and prayerful person. I've seen over three decades of my pastoral ministry with different congregations. This ministry has enhanced my role as a caregiver. Let me share with you my personal experience with my sister who got a stroke a few years ago. She became diabetic that her health conditions had not shown any progress but instead had deteriorated and got serious, which has affected me most since I am the one who is always in constant contact with her and shown more care about her situation. The doctor told me that her condition is getting worse and deteriorating each day. I thought of ministering to her most often while she was still in a nursing home, until her two feet were amputated and she became more helpless and hopeless and became terminally ill. Because of this experience, this has given me an insight of what I can do and how I can be of help to those who are in the same boat as I was, ministering to a terminally ill and dying patient. May this resource manual offer support to those who are engaged in pastoral care.

The following lines are my heartfelt suggestions to all pastoral caregivers so that they can be equipped in ministering to patients as they engage in helping them in their needs, especially those who are in palliative and hospice conditions. Please note that the words "palliative" and "hospice" have strong connotations.

Palliative care can be defined as an approach that improves the quality of life of patients facing life-threatening illnesses, and their families, through the prevention, assessment, and treatment of physical, psychosocial, or spiritual suffering. Palliative care can be delivered along with life-prolonging treatments or as the main focus of care. Palliative care is for all patients with chronic or life-limiting conditions, regardless of life expectancy.

Hospice is a specific type of palliative care that is actually the most intense form of palliative care. Hospice is considered when patients have less than six months of life. Patients agree to enroll in a hospice program and choose not to receive aggressive care. Janice Noort, NP, wrote that "effective and sensitive spiritual care is extremely important for those whom death is imminent. Spiritual needs are very complicated and often difficult to discuss since spirituality and religion are sensitive and personal topics. The role of the spiritual caregiver in palliative care is to be open, listen, observe and when in doubt, ask questions. Performing a spiritual assessment and evaluating for spiritual distress are important aspects of the role of the spiritual caregiver for the dying patient. Essential skills necessary include deep listening and providing a peaceful presence which require human kindness, compassion and caring."[3]

Ministry to the terminally ill and dying patients, as well as to their families, is one of the most sacred privileges of a pastor. It is the time when many people want their pastors to be near them. Our effectiveness in the ministry will be based on how well we have integrated into life what is believed about death and about life.

A hospital chaplain once said, "We have learned that unless pastors are at peace with their mortality and its vast implications, they are not free to accompany others in dying. Fulfillment in death can come only when one's life perspective adequately answers the question of meaning and purpose in the realm of destiny."[9] Basic to the Christian ministry is a life perspective that offers such interpretation. The revelation of Jesus Christ discloses the reality of God's love for us and reveals his concern for man's destiny.

Denial is a natural emotional response. It protects the ego and is necessary if the person needs to distinguish between inevitability of death and the imminence of death. Family and friends are torn between being forced by circumstances to surrender the dying person and being forced by the emotional ties of love to hold on to the patient as long as possible. Loved ones often tell dying persons how much they are needed, the life they can't go on with without them, and they encourage them to fight to the very end. As pastoral caregivers, we face a lot of questions that need answers as we minister to these kinds of patients. Here are some ideas that we need to consider:

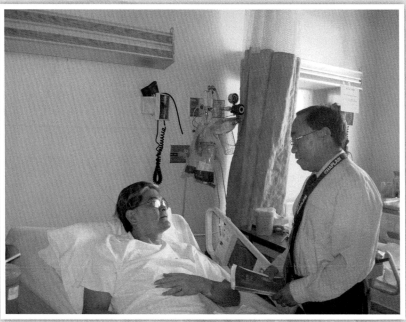

Acts 4:12" 12 Neither is there salvation in any other: for there is none other name under heaven given among men, whereby we must be saved."
Romans 10:13 "13 For whosoever shall call upon the name of the Lord shall be saved."
John 14: 6 "Jesus saith unto him, I am the way , the truth, and the life: no man cometh unto the Father, but by me."

II. The Requisites of the Pastoral Caregivers

A. Pastoral Preparation

A pastor's enactment of his role with hospitalized parishioners plays an important part during the crisis of illness. He must learn to understand patient-physician relationships, coping with illness in the family, as well as family concerns during illness. Providing basic support is essential, just being there and caring while at the same time symbolically representing the love of God. The sharing of the scripture and prayer as well as counseling can refocus values, assist decision making, and affirm relationships, which are very important. A pastor's preparation must also be continuous by participating in a clinical pastoral education (CPE) program. If CPE is unavailable, there are other ways to grow as a helping person during life crises. A senior minister who is willing to be a mentor can be an alternative.

B. Provision of Pastoral Care

It is not uncommon for ministers to be impressed to the point of being intimidated at how concrete and measurable the tasks performed by most health professionals are. In an effort to compensate, I have seen pastors become overly active in hospital visitation, expressing anxiety through attempts at humor, taking dirty laundry home to be washed, or going to a gift shop to buy newspaper. This suggests a lack of clarity in pastoral identity, heightened somewhat by the loss of status and insecurity toward the skilled task performed by others. Few people enter the patient's room with the task of listening to them. Yet feelings and concerns, values, self-image, and faith issues are storming inside, needing to be shared. This is the strength of the pastoral role—to be able to sit and listen with understanding. The patient needs to feel blessed by feeling enough worth that someone would be concerned to hear what the illness experience is like. Self-worth, which is normally defined by doing something or productivity, is unavailable to the patient. Discovering worth is simply elusive, until you have the experience of being listened to with attendant emotions of being accepted and forgiven.

Our ministry to the terminally ill is to be a listener. Simple reflection, a touch, and a listening ear will minister and speak volumes. This skill of listening is hard work, because when done well, the ear is informed by good counseling skills, relevant knowledge, and the wisdom of faith. It is the most active process. The minister cannot count incision stitches or medicines prescribed to measure worth. Being clear about the pastoral role is crucial to the enactment of it, particularly during crisis experiences. I asked some questions to medical persons at UC Davis Medical Center in Sacramento, California, and found answers that are beneficial to our care. Here are their insights and understanding regarding terminally ill patients as well as the people around them.

1. *What are the emotional reactions you see when you tell patients they are terminally ill?*

5

- My experience is that patient and family typically display the various stages of grief—denial, anger, bargaining, depression, and acceptance in addition to anxiety. The stages they go through are not experienced in any particular order. Occasionally patients and/or family remain "stuck" in one stage such as anger or depression and sometimes the stage of acceptance is never attained![3]

- As one could imagine, the reactions of patients are quite varied. Many patients have suspected that they are quite ill and have a very bad illness and are not very surprised by the information. Many other patients, especially patients with young/teenage children are quite despondent and their first response is to think about their children and their needs. Many of those patients become angry and immediately vow to "beat their illness." The third typical reaction is patient is shocked by the news and basically shuts down emotionally and is unable to engage in any more meaningful conversation at that time.

- The most important thing for me to remember is to make sure I have time to be able to deliver the information and be as present for the patient and family as I can be. I never appear rushed. I am prepared to just listen and answer questions. I do not try and deliver too much information as they are usually not in a frame of mind to remember much.[4]

- I see full spectrum of reactions from denial to anger to acute distress/sadness.[1]

2. *How do you prepare the family for the nearing end of their loved ones?*

- I feel it is important the family receive necessary education regarding the dying process and also have the emotional/spiritual support they need during this difficult time. People have many different ideas about the dying process and for many it is their first experience in dealing with death. It is essential that families receive information on what to expect so the mystery associated with death is removed and they understand death is a natural, inevitable process. I encourage questions and make every attempt to provide needed information in a way that can be understood. There are times family members do not want to discuss dying at length and I am respectful of their wishes. I will have the chaplains and social workers get involved for additional support when appropriate.[3]

- The simplest questions to help families are "What are you most concerned about for your loved one?" "What are you or your loved one most worried about?" "What information or questions answered do you need to help you through this process?" "How can I can best help you and your loved one?"[4]

- I try to be frank in my discussion of their loved one's terminal illness. I do not want to give them false hope. I need them to be as best prepared as they can be to handle the upcoming issues. I offer as much emotional support as I can and be sure we fully optimize support for home once patient is discharged.[1]

3. *How do you cope with the stress in dealing with the terminally ill?*

- Palliative care team members are definitely at high risk of developing compassion fatigue due to the associated stress. I find working in a multidisciplinary team with a shared goal helps me cope. Through collaboration and communication, we can be more effective, which helps control stress. As a palliative care team, we also try to focus on team building activities to create a support system for one other. I have found it is also important to develop a sense of self-awareness and practice self-care activities, including exercise, relaxation, socialization with friends/family and reading. I try to acknowledge my limitations and ask for help when I need it. I attempt to maintain a sense of balance in my life and think it's important to keep one's sense of humor![3]

- It is emotionally taxing to deal with the terminal patient and their families. I feel personal sadness for patients and their families. It is important to recognize your own emotion and the vulnerability that you feel in working with such patients. Self-care is the most important thing to help. Taking time for your personal needs whatever they are is important to recharge yourself. It is also important to realize that one cannot fix everything and we should not feel that it is our job to do so, but rather many times it is just important to be present with patient and family, acknowledge the stress, emotion, etc., but not try to fix it.[4]

- I have learned to separate my work from my personal life. Leave the stresses/emotions at work, for work.[1]

4. *How do you handle hostility from family members?*

- I try to remember that the goal is not to prevent a family member from experiencing emotions such as anger, sadness, fear, and loss since these are normal responses. I feel my role is to maintain a trusting therapeutic relationship and safe/supportive environment that allows emotions to be expressed in a positive way if possible. I try to legitimize the appropriateness/normalcy of their reaction and try to explore what is underneath the emotion. I believe it is important to show empathy and explore strengths/coping strategies if possible. I often involve chaplains and social workers if the situation is very emotional.[3]

- Hostility from families is generally not a personal attack on you. They are angry at the diagnosis, situation. They may be in denial about the situation. They may need to blame someone or something for the situation that their loved one is in. I do not internalize their emotion or respond to it. I try to understand what is the driving force behind their emotion. I become a very active listener and spend very little time talking. I do not respond back with any emotion other than sympathy, empathy, and compassion. If the situation becomes too stressful, I will simply excuse myself and offer a time to come back to talk at a more peaceful time.[4]

- Rare for this to happen. Usually, family members are upset that diagnosis was not discovered sooner. They want to blame previous medical providers. Again, I try to offer as much emotional support. Just to be as honest as I can be in my medical assessment and recommendations. Reassure them that the best care possible is being delivered at this time.[1]

5. *What are some resources you give to family?*

- I have a few resources I like to utilize and give to families, which I have found very helpful, including the booklets "Approaching End of Life Together: A Guide for Patients and Caregivers" by Judy Alexander, RN, CHPN, and Martha J. Macri; "A Time To Live: Living with a Life-Threatening Illness" by Barbara Karnes; and "Gone From My Sight: The Dying Experience" by Barbara Karnes.[3]

- I usually do not give specific resources to the family outside of medical follow-up, social services for the home. Appreciate help from discharge planning, social worker, and chaplain.[1]

C. Prayer, Scripture, and Sacraments

Most clergy agree that prayer is a necessary and appropriate part of the pastoral visit. Let us begin with a basic theological foundation of prayer. We affirm first that God is present with us, always seeking healing for us; God doesn't send illness for punishment. Even though all of us know this, it is easy for a person who is ill to revert to superstitious religion, which suggests that this particular affliction may be willed by God. We participate in a world of nature-set free will, which has all kinds of capacity to become destructive. But God does not equal nature. John A. T. Robinson says that "God does not cause the cancer, but God's face may be found in the cancer." This means that God is ever present, always with us, always accessible, always struggling in us, and with us for healing. Our pain is God's pain, as God suffers with us. In fact, it is sometimes worth understanding that the sick and hurting parts of our body are loved by God, unconditionally, just as we are loved by God unconditionally.

The images of prayer are open hands rather than of a clenched fist, of facial muscles relaxing rather than furrowed brows, of deep and restful breathing rather than the gasp of intense supplication. Prayer needs not be a stressful search for God but a nurturing acceptance of God's inexhaustible love. To pray this way may start healing. I believe it is important to pay attention to how the resistance and affirmation of healing function in our own lives and listen to clues of how they are operating in the life and illness of the patient before us. There is a mystery in prayer beyond which none of us can ever fully penetrate. Remember, you are one of the many healers. It is not up to you to be perfect. It is up to you to be a channel for God's healing love to flow through you to the person before you in need. Prayer has a way of opening a door for God's love to flow through us.

When you are with a patient who is chronically ill, hospitalized for a long period, you may have spent time in your visits hearing precious stories of childhood, falling in love, child rearing, and careers. Lift up these memories in prayer for their strength and power.

Another powerful way to share the presence of God with patients is in the reading of scripture. Neither prayer nor scripture should be a substitute for listening and sharing the concerns of the patient. Instead, they are ways to bring comfort and strength, a reminder that none of us is alone, whether a visitor or a patient. You may include in your prayer some scripture references that can meet the variety of needs of the patient. Often the scripture lesson of the past Sunday is good to share. This is a way to connect the patient with the life of the congregation, and you may share your thought as they are related to that passage.

Beyond the sharing of prayers and scriptures, the sacraments offer opportunities for healing mediated through the elemental symbols of faith. The sacraments link the patient with God and the community of faith. Yet it often feels cumbersome to administer the sacrament in the hospital room. Some patients feel that the Communion is a suggestion of a terminal illness, so it is important to determine the patient's wishes and discuss the spirit in which the sacrament is offered. If the patient does wish to have Communion, make sure there is no medical problem in his receiving the elements. Then find out if this is something he wishes to share with family or friends or if he prefers to receive it alone.

If the room is shared with another patient, ask the neighboring patient if he wishes to share the sacrament. Explain your understanding of the openness of the sacrament and respect that patient's preference. Notify the nurses' station what you will be doing and ask that you be not disturbed during that period. Another thing, if patient does not indicate belief in God, you can use nature to make him relate or write some papers about their beliefs or use poems or traditions that they practice. Have them relate to it and listen to what they say about their faith and way of life.

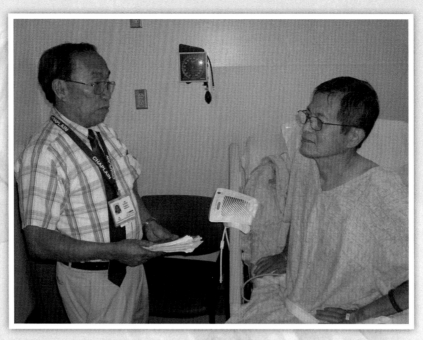

Philippians 4:6-8 " 6. Do not be anxious about anything, but in everything, by prayer and petition, with thanksgiving, present your requests to God. 7 And the peace of God, which transcends all understanding, will guard your hearts and your minds in Christ Jesus. 8 Finally, brothers, whatever is true, whatever is noble, whatever is right, whatever is pure, whatever is lovely, whatever is admirable--if anything is excellent or praiseworthy--think about such things.

III. The Responsibilities of the Pastoral Caregivers

A. Perspective on Period of Time

There is a great challenge for us to be involved in the ministry, especially to the terminally ill or dying patient. The responsibility to be a good minister depends on us. Many illnesses that will shorten life are chronic in nature and extend over a period of several years. This means that much important work must be done prior to death. Bereavement or grief work is a process of adjustment for both acute and chronic phases, often lasting several years or longer beyond the patient's death. Pastoral care begins at the point of diagnosis and is not completed until a reasonable adjustment to the loss has been achieved, usually several years later. The notion of fulfilling the pastoral role through the funeral rituals is superficial, at best.

B. Plans for Living through Serious Illness

Living with and through a serious illness is like running an ultramarathon. It requires thoughtful planning, patience, endurance, and timely support. Although, no one wants to experience it, this type of crisis has the potential of enriching relationships and of being a way into a more meaningful life. It is enough that the potential for goodness resides in what we would all agree is a life event no one would choose to experience. The patient suffering from a terminal illness may experience many behaviors and feelings, which are generally useful for helpers to understand. These feelings include shock, fear, numbness, guilt, anger, depression, lethargy, sadness, self-indulgence, and a host of others. They are normal but not comfortable feelings. Behaviors usually range between the polarities of accepting or denying the realities of the illness. This is normal, and the minister should be prepared for wide variations in the patients' or families' focus on reality. A dying person may want to discuss funeral plans, and sometimes the pastor is the only one willing to talk about the approaching death. Planning for the funeral need not be morbid, for this may be a means of accepting the reality of death, for both the dying person and the family. The patient may want to receive Communion as death draws near, make a public profession of faith and be baptized, or reaffirm his or her faith in preparation for death. If these forms of rituals are acceptable with the patient, you may do so administer with love.

C. Painful Events

Few persons are prepared to live with serious illness or face losing a cherished loved one. Our culture highlights youth, vitality, and health. It cloisters painful events. Most people receive medical treatment and die away from home. As a result, even though everyone experiences death, preparation is rarely part of the normal developmental experience. It is helpful, therefore, for patients and family to have guides, teachers, or counselors to facilitate their way through what amounts to a "foreign country." Health care professional will naturally have opportunities for intervention due to the role of the hospital. The largest periods, however, will be those in the home community, where the pastor is a primary resource.

D. Patients with Bioethical Issues

Another aspect of awareness for the pastor is the possibility of significant bioethical issues in decision making. In the case of terminal illnesses, modern medicine has the ability to sustain life beyond what is meaningful existence. Decisions to withhold or withdraw life-sustaining treatment require careful thought. If the patient is comatose, usually the family must decide. In some states, "natural death" acts recognize express wishes of the patient in the form of a "living will" even if he or she becomes comatose. But the specifics of the law must be observed, and they vary between states having such law. Theological and ethical positions must be considered by the pastor prior to being in a decision-making mode. They must include the ability to support families while minimizing feelings of guilt. The president's commission has produced a series of publications regarding bioethical issues.

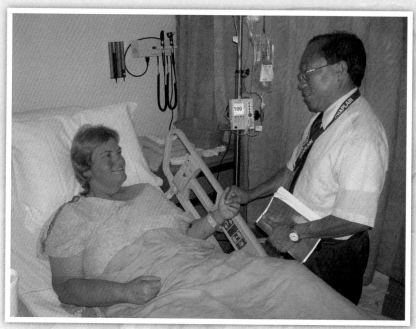

Psalms 37:4-5

3 Trust in the LORD and do good; dwell in the land and enjoy safe pasture. 4 Delight yourself in the LORD and he will give you the desires of your heart. 5 Commit your way to the LORD; trust in him and he will do this:

IV. The Resolutions of the Pastoral Caregivers

A. Prognosis and Diagnosis

When a patient has been told of the diagnosis and prognosis of his illness, he will begin to struggle whether to live or die. It will prompt him to take medication, adhere to therapy, or undergo some surgery. Or will it depress or demoralize him, which will lead to more rapid loss of health, or will it cause him to consider suicide? Will telling them deprive them of happy days without worry, or will it give them the opportunity to bring closer to their life? When they learn that they are so ill, they go through stages, described by Elizabeth Kübler-Ross, which are

(1) *Denial*: "The diagnosis is wrong. The doctors are stupid."

(2) *Anger*: "If only the doctor had run the correct test, I wouldn't be dying now." "If only I had eaten vegetables, I wouldn't have cancer."

(3) *Bargaining*: The dying person may try to bargain for cure and recovery.

(4) *Realistic hope*: If recovery or cure is impossible, the person may come to hope simply that the dying may be delayed or won't give much pain or expense to the family.

(5) *Acceptance*: The person may be able to affirm death as the natural fulfillment of life, the completion of its meaning and purpose; though he may either withdraw from those around him or sense a spirit of peace and equanimity.[2]

Families can accept death when the dying person has been able to find meaning. A dying person can conclude life with a sense of "it is finished" and letting go, knowing that their pilgrimage was not in vain. As a pastor, you can approach them by being positive without expecting that you are going to cheer them up. Be prepared for their feeling of depression, which can be an appropriate reaction to the thought of dying. Your job is to be a manifestation of God's love for and presence to them. When in doubt, try to imagine how Jesus would treat them, and act accordingly. Pray for them.

B. Personal Needs

1. Physical: Persons who are terminally ill experience worsening symptoms. For example, skin conditions, allergies, or spastic colon may worsen. More serious conditions such as ulcerative colitis, lupus, sarcoid, hypertension, and asthma may flare up due to stress in the immune system. Scripture reading is appropriate in line with the physical condition of the patient. Always close in prayer for healing, courage, power, strength, and hope.

2. Emotional: Patients who are dying can be weepy, depressed, or angry. They can say hateful words and hurtful things while at the same time want to be understood. Some who are terminally ill of cancer or AIDS are not open and honest about their condition because of the societal stigma against a person with this disease. They may be embarrassed of a pastoral visit, thinking that they will be rejected. Some are even frightened because of the medical equipment hooked up to them. As a minister, do not act fearful because they might retreat emotionally from you. Do not look shocked because they might conclude that they are closer to the end of their lives than they really are. As a minister of God, you are a representative of God's love. If you make another visit, do not be surprised if the vitality diminishes. The work of dying saps one's energy. So he may be less willing to communicate than at other visits. Respect that. All you need to do is be present; God will do the rest. Pray with the patient if he wishes to but do not insist on it. Allow him to voice his own prayer, if he wishes. Don't be surprised if the prayers are full of anger at whoever caused the illness or at God.

3. *Spiritual:* Spiritually, people with terminal illness have serious questions about God's motives in permitting them to be so ill. Some even hate God, so they don't want to pray, hear about God, or see anyone from the church or a pastor. Many question the existence of God or question the goodness of God—why he permits them to suffer. Some patient wonders if God is punishing them for their past sins by giving them this sickness, so they reject the overtures of pastoral visitors, who are, after all, emissaries of the God whom they question. They may be angry with God and direct these feelings toward the pastoral visitors. Others may be empty, unable to pray, and unable to express their feelings about God. They may feel as if they are in a desert or a wasteland. They may feel too disconsolate or too misunderstood to even hope for someone—especially a pastoral person—who can understand them. At the moment, this is the best time to share the Gospel to patients, reconcile them to God, and let them experience the peace that they need as they come to the end of their journey. You need to prepare the soul of the patients for eternity and assurance of God's love and care by putting their faith on Jesus Christ, who died, was buried, and rose again on the third day. They have to trust Jesus and make him as their Lord and Savior and have that relationship with Jesus and be ready to be with him as soon as God calls them home.

C. Parental Concern

Family members are often anxious, even to the point of being distraught, but still they hope for recovery of the patient. Thus, the usual concerns become magnified under the unfamiliar stresses; the strange sights, sounds, and smell may increase the anxiety and trauma already being experienced by the patient. Death anxiety, generalized apprehension, boredom, loneliness, guilt, denial of reality of their condition, irritability, depression, despair, and resentment are all part of the negativities that are experienced by a terminally ill patient, which parents should be concerned of. As a pastor, show your support. Often pray with them but always ask first if they want to take the lead. Ask if there is anything that you or members of the congregation can do to assist them and their family. You may need to ask more than once. Make sure that you follow through on any promises that you make, especially when you promise for a return visit, to minimize the chance that the family might feel abandoned by the church when they need assistance. We can offer proof of God's love for them not only in words but, more importantly, in actions.

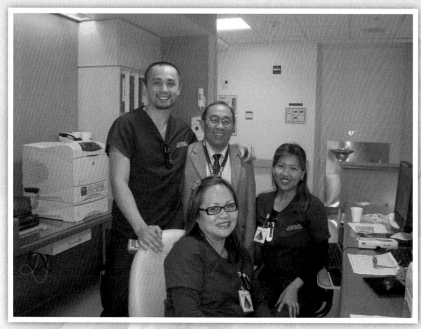

James 5:15-16 "15. And the prayer of faith shall save the sick , and the Lord shall raise him up ; and if he have committed sins, they shall be forgiven him. 16. Confess your faults one to another, and pray one for another, that ye may be healed . The effectual fervent prayer of a righteous man availeth much."

Jeremiah 33:3 "Call unto me, and I will answer thee, and shew thee great and mighty things , which thou knowest not."

Exodus 15:26
"And said , If thou wilt diligently hearken to the voice of the LORD thy God, and wilt do that which is right in his sight, and wilt give ear to his commandments, and keep all his statutes, I will put none of these diseases upon thee, which I have brought upon the Egyptians: for I am the LORD that healeth thee."

V. Conclusion

When ministering to the terminally ill or dying patients, "be a companion to the dying person and family in a very special way." The most important skill for ministering to the dying is the capacity for compassion, which should be developed continually throughout one's ministry. A German pastor who works at a hospital gives guidance: "Words become far less important than simple gestures and a shared silence. Sitting with a family, encouraging them to hold the hand of a loved one or put a cold cloth on a perspiring forehead or to moisten parched lips with water, offering prayer, brief and not prolonged, or making a sign of the cross on a dying person's forehead; spelling a family member who needs to take a break or bringing coffee or soft drinks to refresh the family—each of these thoughtful gestures mean more than a thousand words. At the time of death, supporting them in touching the body and talking to it, protecting their privacy as each close relative may want to say good-bye separately and which might help them cry and crying with them, if the tears are there, will speak profoundly of the pastor's care for them and of the Lord's compassionate love."[8]

Families may appreciate joining hands around the bed of the deceased, along with nurses and friends, for prayer of thanksgiving for the person's life and commendation of the person's keeping. Words of comfort for the family should be included and a brief scripture passage. The pastor should take seriously the dying person's premonitions about his death. They may have dreams in which deceased parents call the dying person to join them. The pastor may help the dying person by encouraging him to tell his life story. Many people can sum up their lives in a few stories from their past. In listening, the pastor can help the dying person find peace, wholeness, completion of life, and acceptance of death.

Be supportive to the family and friends as they grieve and release the dying. Grief causes pain, and the bereaved need understanding, patience, and acceptance. No matter how long a person may anticipate the death of a loved one, the actual moment is still a painful experience, though there may be also a deep sense of relief—both for the self and for the person who died.

During this time of crisis, you can assess and understand their self-image and discover how it affects them. As a pastoral caregiver, you can keep an open communication with the ones left behind. Help them to see the light at the end of the tunnel they are passing through and that there is hope. You are the helper God has called to walk with them through this transition of crisis. Your prayer and support makes a difference in the life of a dying person.

May God richly bless you in this worth-rewarding ministry you are engaged in!

Bibliography

1. Allen Tong, MD, General Medicine, UC Davis Medical Center, Sacramento, CA.

2. Dr. Norman Wright, *Crisis and Trauma Counseling* (Regal Books, 2003).

3. Janice Noort, NP, Palliative Dept., UC Davis Medical Center, Sacramento, CA.

4. John McMillan, MD, Medical Director, UC Davis Hospice, Sacramento, CA.

5. Scott Louis Diering, *Love Your Patients* (Blue Dolphin Publishing, 2004).

6. Peter Kreeft, *Making Sense Out of Suffering* (St. Anthony Messenger Press, 1986).

7. Pat Fosarelli, *Ministering to Ill and Dying Children and their Families* (Liguori Publication, 2003).

8. Helen Fitzgerald, *The Mourning Handbook* (The Fireside Book, 1994).

9. Lawrence D. Reimer and James T. Wagner, *The Hospital Handbook* (Morehouse Publishing, 1984).

Printed in the United States
By Bookmasters